UNDERSTANDING AND ADDRESSING
CHILDREN'S
Grief Issues

UNDERSTANDING AND ADDRESSING
CHILDREN'S
Grief Issues

DAVID A. OPALEWSKI, M.A.
contributions by John Belaski, B.S., M.A.

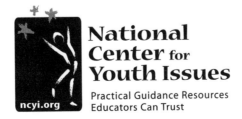

**National
Center for
Youth Issues**

Practical Guidance Resources
Educators Can Trust

P.O. Box 22185 • Chattanooga, TN 37422-2185
423.899.5714 • 800.477.8277
fax:423.899.4547 • www.ncyi.org

P.O. Box 22185
Chattanooga, TN 37422-2185
423.899.5714 • 800.477.8277
fax: 423.899.4547
www.ncyi.org

ISBN: 978-1-931636-47-6
© 2008 National Center for Youth Issues, Chattanooga, TN
All rights reserved.

Written by: Dave Opalewski, M.A.
Contributions by: John Belaski, B.S., M.A.
Cover and Interior Design: Phillip Rodgers
Published by: National Center for Youth Issues

Printed in the United States of America

Table of Contents

About the Authors

Dave Opalewski, M.A,

Dave is the founder and president of Grief Recovery Inc., in Saginaw, Michigan, a consultant and coauthor of *Confronting Death in the School Family, Understanding and Addressing Adolescent Grief Issues* (both published by National Center for Youth Issues) and *Teen Suicide Prevention for Schools and Communities.*

Dave has been in education since 1972. He has also served as an aftercare consultant and grief support group facilitator for a funeral home. He has taught at the elementary, middle, secondary and college levels. Dave is a former At-Risk Coordinator for a K-12 school district and is presently a full-time instructor for Central Michigan University teaching Death and Dying and Suicide Prevention and Adolescent Psychology. He actively participates in professional forums and is highly sought after as a speaker at state and national professional conferences. He has been published several times in professional journals.

During Dave's educational career, he has experienced the death of 28 students and fellow staff members. He was the replacement teacher in a 5th grade classroom for a teacher who was killed in a train-automobile accident.

As a grief-response consultant, Dave is widely sought out by schools to help them establish and implement a tragedy component to their crisis response program.

He can be reached at (989) 249-4362, or by e-mail griefrecovery@chartermi.net or you can visit his website at www.griefrecovery.ws

Contributing Author

John Belaski, B.S., M.A.

John has had an eclectic work career. He has taught on multiple levels of education including community college and university work; is a former business owner and has worked for the Federal Reserve System. John has administered programs and served as an agency director in the human services field—including individual, family and substance abuse counseling.

John is currently co-director of the Safety, Security and Crisis Management Institute, which is a service of Kent Intermediate School District in Grand Rapids, Michigan. He also supervises grants and provides consulting and training services at Kent ISD.

This work done

in dedication

to my wife,

Debbie,

and children

Jeff, Andy and Jenny.

You are all precious

gifts from God.

– Dave

Forward

After the completion of my last book, *Understanding and Addressing Adolescent Grief Issues*, it was my perception that all my major writing projects were complete. I purposely chose not to tackle writing a book on children and grief because unlike *Adolescent Grief Issues*, there is a great wealth of quality information already published. Although I do have a great amount of experience concerning this issue, I did not want to write just another book about an issue I felt, and still feel, is very well addressed by many well-qualified and caring professionals. Also, with the success of *Confronting Death in the School Family*, and *Adolescent Grief Issues* books, I really have no need to tackle this project from a business perspective.

However, literally hundreds of people who have read *Confronting Death* and *Adolescent Grief Issues* have been communicating to me the need for a book on children and grief similar in format. They state that they not only like the format of the other two books, but also like the non-clinical approach, which makes it easy to understand and apply the information provided. Because of these many requests, I organized my thoughts and constructed a non-clinical, informational and practical book for you to better understand, comfort and guide grieving children through the grief process. In the course of this project, I lean on and give credit to the many fine, dedicated people who have worked hard to provide comfort and care to children who are emotionally wounded by events beyond their control.

The following is a result of research, personal experiences, personal mistakes and stories put together to assist adults facing these issues with grieving children. Please be aware, however, that what you have in your heart is far more important than the knowledge that any book can put in your head.

Introduction

I want to take this opportunity to share with you about my wife, Debbie, and our two sons, Jeff and Andy. My wife is a former widow. We started dating five years after the death of her husband Larry. Jeff, the oldest boy, was 14 months old and Debbie was two months pregnant with Andy at the time Larry died. Although this was an extremely difficult time for Debbie, I wish to focus on how Larry's death affected the two young boys.

According to Debbie, "There is no question that Jeff, at 14 months old, grieved the death of his father. I could tell he missed his dad and was very sad but I couldn't explain the death to him. The day Larry died, a part of Jeff also died. The smile that only his father could bring out in him was gone and has never been seen again. Larry had a favorite red sweater that he wore often. Shortly after his death, Jeff saw a man similar in size of Larry wearing a red sweater. Jeff was sitting in his car seat and began to cry uncontrollably and pointed to the man while trying to break out of his car seat. Jeff certainly did grieve the death of his father, even though he was just over one year old."

On my second date with Debbie, we took the boys to an ice cream store. While we were eating our ice cream, Andy (then five years old) said to me, "My dad loved Jeff but he didn't love me." Once Debbie and I were over our astonishment, I asked Andy why he felt his dad didn't love him. Andy replied, "because he was alive for Jeff but died before I was born." The forlorn look on Andy's face brought tears to our eyes. This boy, only two months in the womb when his father died, was definitely grieving the death of his father.

Debbie tells another very compelling story supporting the fact that young children do indeed grieve the death of a loved one. "I was shopping at the mall with the two boys. Jeff was five years old and Andy was almost three years old. The boys saw the water fountain at the center of the mall and asked if they could throw a penny into the fountain. I gave them each a penny and told them to make a wish before they threw their penny into the water. They closed their eyes, made their wish and both threw their penny into the water. Then they turned to me and asked if I wanted to know what they wished for. I told them that it was their secret wish. Ignoring my comment, Jeff told me that he wished for a new dad. Andy then said, "me too!" That really brought tears to my eyes and an ache in my heart. From my experience as a widow with two young children, I have no doubt that children, even very young children, grieve the loss of a loved one."

As an aftercare consultant in a funeral home for three years and a grief support group facilitator, I have seen and heard many similar stories demonstrating that young children do indeed grieve. It is also common knowledge that these children are at a higher risk for depression as they grow. When they become adolescents, they are at a much higher risk for suicidal and other risk-taking behaviors. The American Psychiatric Association states that, "The death of a parent before age 8 puts the adolescent at higher risk for suicide attempts." Many experts also claim that most of these children will go through attachment disorder sometime in their lives. Andy went through attachment disorder at a young age while Jeff went through it later in adolescence. Even though I adopted the boys, and have a very loving relationship with them, they still went through attachment disorder even though they've called me dad from the time we announced our engagement.

In summary: a child who experiences the death of a parent, sibling or other close loved one *does indeed grieve*. These grieving children must have the loving guidance of an adult if they are to grow to be emotionally healthy. It is the goal of this book to help you as you comfort, care and guide a child through this difficult process.

Chapter 1

Facts About Children and Grief

Chapter One

Facts About Children and Grief

The National Center for Health Statistics in a recent survey states that one in every seven children loses someone close to them by death before the age of ten. This means literally thousands of young children experience the expected or unexpected death of parents, siblings, grandparents or other loved ones. In addition to those who experience the death of a sibling or parent, there are countless friends, classmates and relatives of these children who encounter grief for the first time in their young lives. All too often these children are the "forgotten grievers" and are expected to simply get on with life.

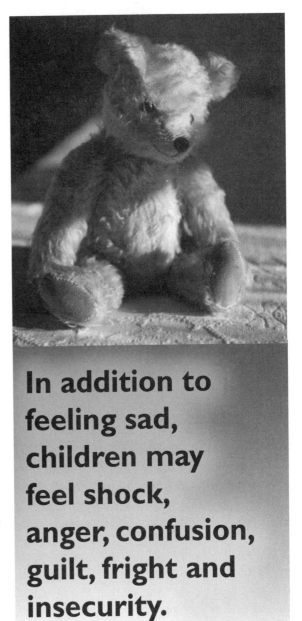

Special Challenges

Young children generally face more challenges than adults in understanding and grieving a loss. In addition to feeling sad, children may feel shock, anger, confusion, guilt, fright and insecurity. In contrast to adults, children face these challenges without the benefit of life experiences and emotional maturity to deal with these feelings.

In addition to feeling sad, children may feel shock, anger, confusion, guilt, fright and insecurity.

Bouncing In and Out of Grief

In one of my many experiences as an aftercare consultant for a funeral home caring for families of the deceased, a young child (about 5 years old) came to the visitation for his deceased grandfather. After he had a healthy cry, he went to the other end of the emotional spectrum. He was told that he and his family were going to McDonald's® for dinner, before the evening visiting hour at the funeral home. The young boy was elated that he was going to get a "Happy Meal®" at McDonald's® and he was not shy about telling visitors where he was going for dinner. This is very normal behavior for a young child. Children usually bounce in and out of grief, crying one moment and laughing the next. This young boy had another healthy cry just before leaving the funeral home to go to McDonald's®. This is very confusing for children because they don't understand why they bounce in and out of grief so

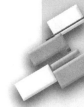

quickly. It is also confusing for most adults in trying to understand the child's emotional reactions and, therefore, the needs of the grieving child.

Behavior

Adults, because of their established vocabulary, can usually connect words with feelings. Children may be too young to connect words with feelings. Thus, the way children can best express themselves is through their behavior. One example is they may become aggressive or hurt themselves as a way of relieving pain they can't express. Others, as a result of fear, may become withdrawn, unwilling to share thoughts and feelings, harboring their fears inside.

Play

In 1988, I was a Physical Education teacher in an elementary school. A close friend of mine for 16 years was one of the 5th grade teachers. My friend was killed in a car accident on a Friday evening in February. I was the replacement teacher in his classroom the following Monday morning. This was an experience in life you would never want to sign up for. However, after going through this difficulty, I learned a great deal about helping grieving children I would not have learned by doing research. The children taught me more than I could have ever imagined. While in this circumstance, my approach toward the children was to express how I was feeling about the tragedy to legitimize their feelings. As a result, the children saw me as more than their teacher—they saw me as a human being also mourning this loss along with them. They also taught me that *grief shared is grief diminished*. In sharing our grief, we encouraged each other. However, this may not always be the best approach. The children may need someone to provide a high degree of stability at this time. Sharing how you are impacted by the tragedy may hinder efforts to provide stability. The adult in charge must make this decision.

That particular Monday morning, the playground supervisors were very upset when they discovered a group of first grade students in our school were acting out during play how they perceived this tragedy had occurred. Experts agree that this is normal and healthy behavior if the children choose to do this on their own, without any prompting from adults. This type of play usually includes their feelings and understanding of the tragedy. In instances where there is a high degree of volatility or hysteria, I highly recommend that if children indicate that they do want to act out what happened, they do so under the supervision of a professional.

Behavior and play become one of the few outlets children have when they lack life experiences in the understanding of a tragedy and how it fits into everyday life. Remember, as stated before, they usually do not have a vocabulary to connect words and feelings. With this in mind, children need physical comfort, sympathy, compassion and an opportunity to express themselves in their own way far more than they need advice. I will expand more on this idea in the upcoming chapters.

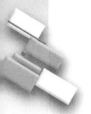

Understanding and Addressing Children's Grief Issues
© National Center For Youth Issues • www.ncyi.org • 1-800-477-8277
Please refer to page 4 for duplication information

Age Considerations

Before I discuss specific age considerations of the child, I wish to express the fact that grief is a unique experience to all individuals, including children. I do not believe in the theory that grieving children of a certain age group grieve in a certain way. I believe that each child will, in some phase of the grief journey, respond in an atypical and unique manner. However, there are times when a peer group's influence will impact children, causing their behaviors to fall into typical patterns. Although we do find some general typical grief responses relative to age, caring adults must afford the opportunity to the grieving child to teach us what grief is like for him.

Common Grief Responses and Patterns

Please bear in mind that while I am attempting to list typical patterns, the uniqueness with which people experience grief may not show up on my lists.

Baby to Age Two – Increased crying, thumb sucking, fussier, sleep more or less, eat more or less.

Preschoolers - ages 3 to 6 – May be frightened and may not understand their feelings. They usually cannot verbalize what is going on inside them. They may ask some questions about the death over and over again. They also may act out the death through play. Regression to thumb sucking, losing potty training and baby talk are common. They usually don't understand the permanence of death.

Ages 6 to 9 – Many experts state that children in this age group primarily express their grief through play. Many may appear to misbehave or act in such a way that adults perceive their actions as misbehavior. This may occur because of children's confusion over how to handle their grief feelings and, in many cases, their actions may not really constitute misbehavior at all. Their questions may revolve around curiosity about the decomposition of the body and the biological process of death. They also may believe the person may be alive in the grave. The permanence of death is still very difficult to comprehend.

Ages 9 to 12 – At this age children are developing a better understanding of death. They are usually ready for more information or answers to these questions:

- Why did the death happen?

- What is and what happens at a funeral?

- What is the reason for a funeral?

- Will others they love die?

- What will happen to them if a parent or both parents die?

As caring adults, our role is to help children grieve. We need to support and educate them, not protect them from grief. We must realize that grief is the solution, not the problem. Unfortunately, the child must be allowed to feel his pain if he is going to heal. Rather than advice, the greater needs of the child are physical comfort, sympathy and compassion.

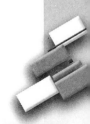

chapter

2

Building a Foundation

Chapter Two

Building A Foundation

Contributed by John Belaski

Sometimes when I consider the enormity of grief and loss issues that many young children face, I feel (as I imagine they do) overwhelmed by it all. I have tried to consider just what it is that I, as a relatively competent and caring adult, can offer them that will make it a little easier to deal with. After all, I have been trained in a helping profession (particularly in the field of Crisis Response) and I have a fair amount of life experience as well. Along with that thought comes the desire to suggest things to educators and parents that will provide some resources and techniques that will help them lighten the load of the young ones they walk with in this life.

Never Too Late

Recently, in an almost accidental way, I stumbled across one concept that resonated with me and led to a few other potentially useful ideas. It started with a phone call I finally made to an acquaintance who had suffered a great loss in her family. I had felt incapable of responding to the enormity of the loss and consequently did not initially call or visit the family. Perhaps it was because I knew and liked the family that I found it very hard to respond in a way that I might have responded to in a "professional" situation. Time passed and I remained immobile with regard to a caring and meaningful response. Even though I really cared about this family, in most situations grieving people, including children, will perceive this absence of response as indifference. Fortunately, I had the opportunity to sit in on a class with a colleague and friend who addressed this very issue. In this class Rabbi Al Lewis reflected on the reality that a hole in the fabric of your life never really goes away. He said that support is always needed and there is never a time when it is "too late." Anniversaries, birthdays and so many other events remind people of their losses and offer myriad points in time when we can be caring and nurturing. I finally had a way to offer support in the form of that late but heartfelt call.

Establishing Quality Relationships

In a larger sense, if we look at the "enormity of the loss" incurred by a grieving child, one possible answer to their need is to "BE THERE" for them in whatever form and in whatever time frame they need. It is important to note that this is not only a potential "response" to their needs after a tragedy, but we really should see this as a "before" as well as an "after" action. If we make a commitment to be involved in children's lives and we interact, communicate, problem solve, have fun and "BE THERE" for them as they move through their lives, we can be of greater assistance after a tragedy. Children need a quantity of quality time from the adults in their lives.

One Family's Story

An example of a person "BEING THERE" for a child fell into my lap as I was beginning to write the material for this chapter. I was driving home from work and heard part of a program on the radio that dealt with this same topic. As I became aware that the ideas being discussed were related to this issue, I heard a mother describing some of what her family did in working through the impending and inevitable death of her husband.

They were a family that discussed issues very openly, so her young son was aware that his father was dying. As I recall the interactions in the family, things went as smoothly as one could hope until the young boy, unexpectedly and quite out of character, began to be very hostile and negative towards babies. The mother was very sensitive and attuned to her child's needs, so she took note of the change in him very quickly.

Even though she made prodigious and caring efforts to explore this behavior with her son, it took her a long time to figure it out. Finally her efforts were rewarded with success. She discovered that at some point in the past, a well-meaning adult had talked about the concept that there is an order to our lives such that all human life passes in time but is replaced by other souls who enter the world. As I heard the concept, I thought that perhaps for some people that thought could be comforting. There is a sense of orderliness and larger purpose to death and new life in that context. However, that is not the way this sensitive young child saw the situation.

After hearing this idea, the young child likely followed a line of reasoning which suggested that if new babies come into the world to take the place of older people (like his dad) who were leaving, then if the new babies did not come along, his dad might not have to leave.

The Lesson

I cite this beautiful story for several reasons. First, the mother was truly there for her child and beautifully worked through this difficult situation. It was not easy and took time and sensitivity that ultimately resulted in a positive outcome. Imagine the long-term (and even the short-term) possibilities if no one had been there to hear, understand and help sort things out with this child. Secondly, we have to be truly careful and aware of the possible implications of the way we explain issues to young people when we are helping them deal with grief and loss. That has been referred to elsewhere in this book, but this example underscores it in a useful and poignant way.

Finally, as I reflect on the incident mentioned above, it occurs to me that we can and should expand the idea of who responds to the grief of a young child, beyond the people most closely involved, like the mother I cited above. We need to take the concept of support and understanding to another level.

We can create the type of environment where we are not just available to young people as individuals but where we do so as an entire community.

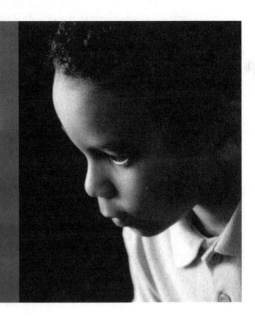

We can create the type of **environment** where we are not just available to young people as individuals but where we do so as an entire **community**. We need to look at all children as all of **our** children. We need to "BE THERE" for youth, whether we have children or not, whether we are in the helping professions or in business, or whether we are "trained" in dealing with crisis situations or not.

Building CommUNITY

In our society, many of us seem to have abdicated our duty as a friend, neighbor or community member. Today, we have people who "know" and have "friends" in other states and countries with whom they interact electronically through the internet, yet they hardly know or interact with their own neighbors (to say nothing of their neighbor's children). Perhaps as we consider ways that we can recognize and assist young children in dealing with the powerful issues of grief and loss, we can recognize that these issues need the COMMUNITY to respond if we are to be maximally effective in our efforts.

In response to these ideas, I have heard people say that they do not have the training or that these things are better left to the professionals or to a minister. My response is that we have left too much to the professionals. There are not enough of them to be available in the depth and at the times we need them most. We must work with them. In assisting and supporting each other, we will do a far better job in coping with the needs of our young people than if either group tries to do it alone.

Connecting the Community

As a final point in this chapter, I would like to give you another illustration of why I am making the suggestion that we need the community to be involved with kids **_before_** AND **_after_** any tragedy that requires us to assist young people with grief and loss needs. I am old enough that I remember a time when the community was there for its members young and old. There was no grief, loss or "debriefing" training available. The field did not even exist as a separate professional discipline. Mostly due to affordability, therapy and counseling were not readily available to the average person.

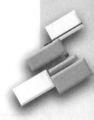

Work from your

HEART

and trust it.

Join with others and

ENCOURAGE

others to do the same.

As a youth I can remember that when a serious or tragic situation occurred, our local church tolled the bells in a particular manner to inform us of its occurrence. Many of us did not have phones or, if we did, they were often eight-party lines that were not easily accessible because they were in use. Private lines were expensive and not always available even if you could afford one. We simply walked down to the church to find out what was happening. In doing so, we met with other friends, neighbors and relatives. This type of response became a community response. We were there for each other.

My home town had a lot of industrial plants, and factory whistles served a similar function. If you heard a particular type of whistle, you knew that it was not a shift change or the noon whistle. You recognized that some serious event had occurred and would travel to the plant to find out what happened or, in some cases, to help in any way that you could. I can remember helping with fire hoses on more than one occasion. Once again, the response was a community response. We knew who was affected. We also knew in what way and to what degree both during and after the event. We rallied as a community to assist and support those in need.

Of course, I am not saying that we should (or can) go back to whistles or church bells, but we can restore our involvement with each other and re-establish our community connections. This is particularly important with our young people. We often say that the youth are our future - and they are - but are we doing anything as a community to help them along, especially in dealing with loss, tragedy and grief and loss issues? Are we looking at this as a pre- and post-set of activities rather than just rallying to someone after something goes wrong in their lives? **Pro-action can be just as effective as re-action in dealing with these issues**.

Building Assets

Let me wrap up with a few specific thoughts. Young people need you, so get involved in the ways we have suggested throughout this book. Work from your heart and trust it. Join with others and encourage others to do the same. Finally, take a serious look at ways of building strength, resiliency and assets in our young people. There are many ways of promoting positive youth development that will result in our young people being in a better position to weather the tragedies and difficulties they will encounter in life.

A few very specific ways you can accomplish what is being suggested here is to become involved in mentoring, tutoring, coaching (academically and in sports) and generally to become involved in building assets in youth (and I do not refer to financial ones). The Search Institute in Minneapolis has developed a list of 40 internal and external developmental assets that are needed by our young people to thrive and survive. You can visit their website at http://www.search-institute.org/ to view the full list. Get involved with your church, school, city and neighborhood in helping develop more of these assets in our young people. You, our youth and communities, to say nothing of our future, will be better if you do so. Most important, though, is that if you implement such actions, young people will cope better with tragedy and grief and loss issues than they do now. This will be true in part because you (and the community) will be there for them, but also because in helping them develop more assets, they will be better able to cope even when you are not there.

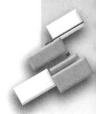

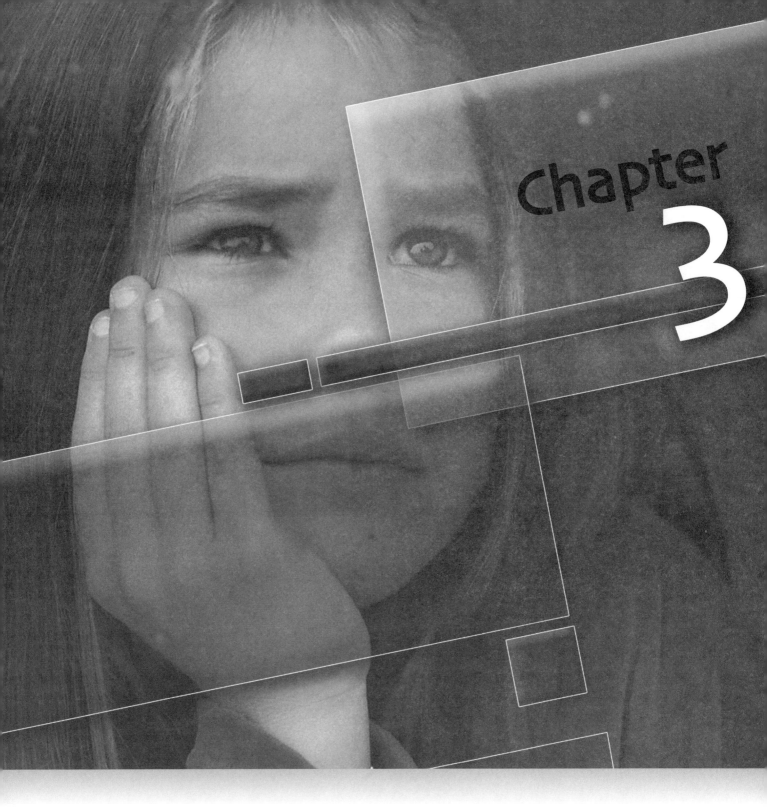

Talking to Children About Death

Chapter Three
Talking to Children About Death

A child today is all too aware of the reality of death, perhaps more than adults realize. At a young age children are confronted with that instance when life no longer exists: a pet dies, grandpa dies, a funeral procession passes by and, of course, the influence of television. When a death does occur, many adults imagine that the fact of death is beyond the child's comprehension or that they need to protect the child from the pain they themselves feel. Both assumptions are wrong and deprive the child of the opportunity to share his grief and learn coping mechanisms from it.

What if I Don't Know What to Say?

No person has all the answers about why a person dies suddenly in an accident or contracts a deadly disease, lingers and then dies. However, not knowing what to say doesn't excuse the adult from the responsibility to share with the child what he does know and understand about the situation. There is no excuse in leaving the bewildered child to muddle through the mess by herself. The wise adult will place herself in a position to receive insight from the grieving child. The wise adult also listens to the child. When the adult does most of the talking, she is not giving enough opportunity to the child to express her feelings and to ask questions. Adults should encourage children to share with them what they feel, think and know about the death. Answering questions in the spirit in which they are asked is key to keeping the communication door open. The communication door is more likely to be kept open if you don't teach the child by your actions that you are the expert who has the final answers the child must accept. You may refer to *Common Grief Responses and Patterns* (p.19) to better understand the child's reaction before considering your response.

The best thing we can say to a child when we don't know the answer to a question is, "I don't know." This communicates a sense of honesty to the child and a willingness of the adult to attempt to get to the child's level of understanding. If the child acts surprised that you don't know, you may say something like this:

"Are you surprised that I don't know everything about death? Please don't be. We can still talk about it. You can learn from me and I can learn from you. We can help each other."

This wise adult is now poised to learn along with the child as they both move through the grief process.

Some Common Adult Mistakes

The following is a list of a few common mistakes I witnessed in my experiences as an aftercare consultant and a grief support group facilitator. Please note that this not a complete list. You may be able to add one or two to the list yourself.

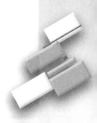

1 ***An Aunt to a Young Boy*** – "Don't feel bad, Freddy. God took your father because He needed him more than you did." Although the motives of this aunt I believe were pure, because she was trying to make Freddy feel better, she made three critical mistakes. First of all, she told Freddy not to feel bad. Why shouldn't Freddy feel bad on the night before his father's funeral? Why shouldn't he be entitled to honest feelings of pain, loss and anger? Second, she spoke to Freddy in terms of God taking his father away. This statement will likely make Freddy resentful of God and less open to the comfort that religion can and does bring to people of all ages. Third, and most critical of all, she suggested that God needed Freddy's father more than he did. I believe she was trying to communicate to Freddy that his father's death was not meaningless and I commend her for her purpose. However, what Freddy heard was that if he only needed his father more, God would not have taken him. In other words, He didn't need him enough and that is why he died. This statement may compound the guilt Freddy is already feeling. It is also important that parents, teachers, counselors and friends are sensitive to the religious viewpoints the child is being taught at home.

2 ***I Know How You Feel*** – When we tell anyone who is grieving the death of a loved one "I know how you feel," we are actually telling them that they can't talk to us, because they know we *don't* know how they feel (including children). Grief is a unique experience for every human being. We don't know how they feel and we anger and/or confuse the grieving person when we say we do. We can say, however, "I have had a similar experience and I have a small inkling of what you may be feeling," or, better yet, "I don't know how you feel but you can tell me." Remember: comfort, care, compassion, listening and understanding are usually the most important needs of the grieving person at this time.

3 ***Minimizing the Loss*** – This is the most common mistake I have witnessed. Examples of minimizing are, "At least you have your brother" (said to a girl who lost her sister in a car accident), or "Your mother is a wonderful, strong and loving person. Focus on how blessed you are to have her" (said to a young girl who lost her father to cancer). Once again, these adults did care and had pure motives. I believe that they were trying to communicate to the child that "all is not bad." They were trying to get the grieving child to focus on the positives. However, a tragedy is a tragedy. We can't fix it and should not try to fix it. Minimizing the loss angers and/or confuses grieving children and adults alike. We also continue to heap guilt upon the grieving child when we try to minimize their loss. When the child feels so bad, he gets more confused about his feelings when some caring adult suggests that "it isn't so bad."

4 ***The Extra Responsibility Role*** – This is a situation when a well-meaning adult says to a young boy who just lost his father, "You have to be the man of the house and take care of your mother and sister." Or it can be vice-versa, with a daughter taking care of her father and brother. The adult may be trying to build the child's self-esteem by saying this, giving her the confidence that she can get through this tragedy. Once again, good intentions but wrong approach. Think about this: the child has just lost a parent, is frightened and possibly angry, and you tell him or her that they will have a very important added responsibility in the household. Here is a child shaken by her loss, and not knowing if she can cope in addition to being the key person running things in the household.

5 ***Answering Questions or Giving Explanations About Death By Using Fairy Tales*** – Although I applaud the effort of the adult to take the time to talk with the child, ***I do not suggest the use of fairy tales.*** Does this prepare the child for life realities? It is not a good

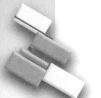

idea to cover up with fiction what you may someday have to repudiate. There are no greater needs for a child at this trying time than trust and truth.

I stress that the above five situations are incomplete. Time and space prevent me from sharing with you most of the wrong things said to children by caring, well-intentioned adults. More suggestions are listed below:

- Don't give them unhealthy explanations about death (Dad went on a long journey).

- Don't say that "They are sleeping now." There is a major difference between sleep and death. The child may be afraid to go to sleep, have nightmares, or both.

- Don't push your theological beliefs on the child.

- Don't force the child to talk about the death if he is unwilling to talk at that time. Communicate to the child that you will check with him from time to time concerning talking about the tragedy. Don't say, "When you want to talk, just let me know." Chances are slim the child will seek you out.

- Let the child go to the funeral home if she desires to do so. Prepare her for what she is going to see at the funeral home (people crying, laughing, the deceased person in the casket, etc.) and don't just drop off the child at the funeral home. Go in with her. Also, if the child wants to attend the funeral, prepare her for what she will probably experience at the funeral. If possible, go with her or have her go with one of her friend's parents.

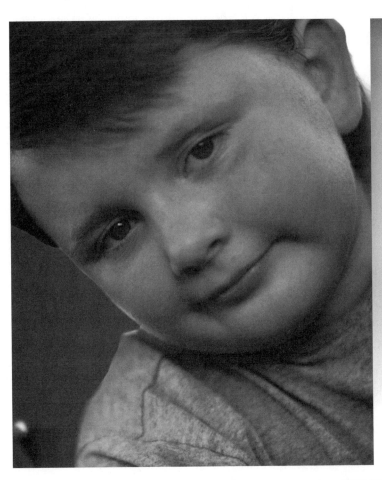

There are no greater needs for a child at this trying time than trust and truth.

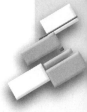

What Adults Can Do

The caring adult must first get in touch with her own feelings about the death.

- Remember, children do not think like adults, so try to enter the child's world. Provide opportunities for expression, such as helping them to construct a sympathy card, write a letter, draw pictures, etc.

- Listen. When adults do most of the talking, they are not providing the opportunity for the child to express his inner feelings.

- Offer assurance, then value and trust the uniqueness of the child's expression.

- Offer opportunities for the child to commemorate the deceased person.

- Share in a real way. When there are no words to say, use a gentle touch on the shoulder. If appropriate, a hug communicates to the child that you will be there for him when he needs to talk.

If the tragedy also traumatizes the adult because of past situations, or he is too close to the tragedy, it may be a good idea for him to excuse himself from the situation. It is okay to do this. The adult must be able to function in a stable manner in this situation. An example of this situation comes from a friend of mine who is a crisis team curriculum coordinator in a different county. He shares about a mother and her two children getting killed in a car accident during the Thanksgiving holiday. The minister who was assigned to the funeral was very close to the family. The two children were enrolled in his church daycare. Upon his arrival to the daycare, he found the minister so wounded by the tragedy that he was virtually non-functional in serving the family and friends of the deceased. In this situation, it was not only okay for the minister to back away from the situation, it was in the best interest of all involved.

Suggestions for Discussing a Tragedy with a Child

The following is a list of suggestions for the caring adult to consider when discussing a tragedy with a child:

- Stop… breathe… calm yourself.
- Think about what you want to say before you sit down with the child.
- Think about how the child may understand your explanations.
- Use short sentences and age-appropriate vocabulary.
- Do not promise anything you can't deliver.
- Encourage the expression of all feelings.
- Listen to their questions.
- Include children in closure rituals.
- Remember: grief is a process, not a time limited event.

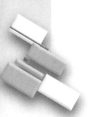

Explaining the Sudden Death of a Sibling, Classmate, Friend or Cousin

The sudden death of another child, whether sibling, friend, cousin or classmate, publicized in the media can be very scary for the child. It introduces into the child's world a sense of vulnerability. This makes the child realize that something painful and scary can happen to someone his age. In discussing these situations with a child or group of children, four important points need to be stressed:

1 When discussing death with children, the adult must communicate to the child that she doesn't have all the answers.

2 The accident that happened was rare. It hardly ever happens. That is why it is on TV or in the newspaper. Almost all the time, when children get sick they get well, or when children get out of their parents' car and walk across the street to school, they do it safely. On very rare occasions, a child becomes incurably ill and dies. When this happens, everybody is very surprised and very sad.

3 What happened to Tommy was not a punishment for his being bad. "If you are remembering that Tommy did something a little naughty a few days ago, and yesterday he became suddenly sick and died, it doesn't mean that if you sometimes do the same thing, something bad is going to happen to you. Tommy didn't get sick because he was a bad boy and deserved to get sick. He deserved to live, play and have fun. This terrible, unexplainable thing just happened."

4 We should not try to "fix" the problem. I facilitate a grief support group for young adolescents. This past year, one of the group members made a statement that I will never forget. He said, "You know what I like about this group Mr. O ?" I said, "No, what do you like the most Chris?" He stated, "You don't try to fix us." I think he was trying to communicate to me several key components discussed in this chapter.

Remember, in caring for children during their grief, it should be our objective to help them grow in their coping skills and **_not_** give them ours.

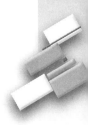

Chapter 4

Explaining Suicide to Children

Chapter Four

Explaining Suicide to Children

There is little doubt that one of the most difficult situations an adult must face is discussing a suicidal incident with a young child. In my experience as a grief support group facilitator, I have spoken with several adults who were in this situation and chose not to discuss it with their children. In most of these cases, the children eventually found out about the incident from other sources. The question one must ask is, from whom is it better for your child to hear such information? Is it better coming from you, where you can influence the situation and give comfort, or from other sources, such as other children, where the situation stands to be embellished or inappropriately explained?

3rd Grade Teacher Commits Suicide

Several years ago at a neighboring school, a third grade teacher attempted and completed a suicide. Administrators were debating what to tell the teacher's students, as well as the entire student body. Time has proven that the administrators made the correct choice in informing the students that their teacher took his life. The administration did so in a very sensitive, sympathetic, and non-judgmental manner.

The children were told that their teacher was very sick with an illness called depression. It was then explained, on their level, how depression makes a person feel and see things far differently than a person who does not have depression. They gave examples. Also, they told the children that people who are depressed can get help and get better. One of the first questions to surface was, "Why did their teacher choose not to get help?" This question received an honest answer, such as, "We don't know. There can be many reasons why Mr. _____ did not get help, but we really don't know for sure. Maybe he was so confused he didn't realize that he could get help." Additional questions were asked by the students and answered in the spirit in which they were asked at an age-appropriate level.

Great Job!

Personally, I think this school administration did a great job of handling this situation. They met the challenge head on. I will list some of the key things this school did that were very appropriate and effective:

- After securing permission from the deceased person's family to announce the death as a suicide, they did so in a classroom setting.

- The school used their own personnel to speak to the students. My research and experiences prove beyond a shadow of a doubt, that the people the students want to talk to after a tragedy such as this are the people they see every day at school and with whom they have established relationships. However, I highly recommend that if you do have support services in your community, or a community crisis team, they be available to support the staff as they reach

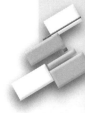

out to the students. Also, if during the crisis the staff becomes too overwhelmed, the support staff is on hand to help.

- The school did not use a professional that the students didn't know.

- They were honest, sensitive, caring, compassionate and non-judgmental.

- When they didn't know the answer to a question, they said, "We don't know." They did not speculate on answers.

- They dispelled guilt. They stressed that no one was the cause of why it happened.

- First, they communicated how they were going to approach this incident with the parents of all the students in the school then they gave the parents some direction and encouraged them to talk to their children about the tragedy. They also allowed parents to call them if they had questions or needed assistance in helping their children.

- The replacement teacher came from the present staff in the building. I don't believe that hiring a stranger is fair to either the students or the teacher. However, in some situations no such person on staff may be available for this assignment. The staff may also be so impacted by the tragedy that no one can fill this role. In this case, support needs to be in place for the replacement teacher as well as the students. In this case, the community crisis team or other community support services will play a critical role.

Exception to the Rule

Unfortunately, the true story I just described is the exception, not the rule in our schools and society. Most think that talking about suicide puts ideas into kids' heads. The American Association of Suicidology dismisses this myth. They state, "Suicide is preventable and the number one preventative measure is to talk about it." It is easy to see, with the growing number of suicides in our country each year, that "*not talking about it*" clearly isn't working. Also, if the child does eventually find out (most do) and knows that you know, what have you actually communicated to the child? The answer to this question is probably that you don't want to talk to the child about this situation. This can be perceived by the child as dishonesty on the part of the parent or a sense that, "It is not worth the effort for my parents to talk to me about the suicide."

> "Suicide is preventable, and the number one preventative measure is to talk about it."

Adult to Child

Let's take a look at a hypothetical situation where someone close to you and your child has completed suicide. As a parent, you sense a strong need to discuss this situation with your child. The following exchange is certainly not perfect nor complete but can give you some useful guidelines when you sit down with your child to talk with him.

- First, make sure you positively know the facts of what happened.

- Timing is important. You need to tell your child before he may hear it from other sources. The best general guideline is to inform as soon as possible.

- Sit down with the child close to you. One of the best ways is to sit across from each other so eye contact can be made and you can touch each other. Your child usually will need hugs or other hypersensitive touch.

- Tell your child, "I have something very sad to tell you and you may feel like crying. You may also feel confused, sad and angry. Crying is okay." You may also say "I may cry and if I do, I will need a hug." This will help the child see your care and compassion. Remember, grief shared is grief diminished.

- Make sure you use the word died along with suicide. Try not to give too much detail as to how the person committed the act.

- One question that will usually come up is, "How did Grandpa die?" Your response may be something like this: "Sometimes we don't understand why people die in a certain way. When someone has cancer or dies in a car accident, we understand it more. But sometimes people do it to themselves. When this happens we say it is suicide. Many times when people do this they have a sickness in the mind that causes them to do this. They are confused, very sad and feel like everything is hopeless. They have it, you don't, I don't. It is hard to understand and it has nothing to do with you or me. I didn't and you didn't do anything to cause this."

- Provide an opportunity for your child to come back and talk with you if he feels bad about the death.

- Your child may demand more of the details. You should give them in simple form without going into great detail. Don't give more information than was asked for.

Remember, grief shared is grief diminished.

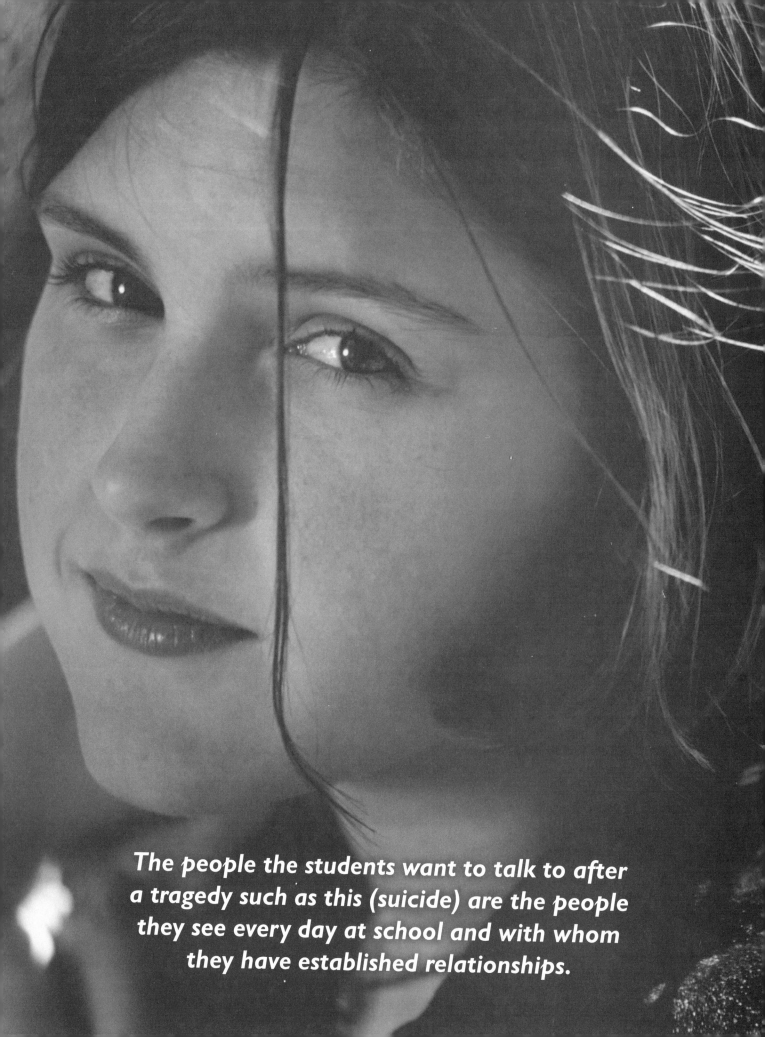

The people the students want to talk to after a tragedy such as this (suicide) are the people they see every day at school and with whom they have established relationships.

- Make sure your child knows that suicide is the act of killing yourself so that your body doesn't work anymore. You may go on to say, "People do this when they feel very sad and feel that life is not worth living. People can often get help, though. Doctors are now very good at helping these people so they feel better."

- If your child asks how he did it, he needs to know, but spare the graphic details.

- Always be honest, because children know when they are being lied to.

- Emphasize that suicide is always a mistake because people can get help.

- Dispel myths.

- Your child may remark, "I thought Grandpa loved me. How could he do this to me?", If so, you could reply that, "Grandpa did love you very much. Because of his depression, or illness in his mind, he couldn't think clearly and his thoughts were mixed up."

If you are honest and sensitively direct, your child will know that he can count on you. This sense of security is of the utmost importance to the child during this scary, confusing time. Although we must stress that suicide is never the answer, it is also important to show sympathy and compassion, not social and spiritual judgment.

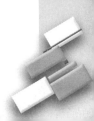

Chapter 5

A Death in the Family

Chapter Five

A Death in the Family

When death impacts a family, everyone has a great need to feel understood, yet a natural incapacity to be understanding. Catholic Family Services and Lutheran Family Services both tell us that "62% of marriages will end in divorce within two years after the death of a child." This is an extremely difficult time for even the best of families.

Anticipated death

Anticipated deaths are considered by many to be "good deaths" because the fore-warning provides loved ones the chance to come to terms with the situation before the inevitable occurs. People supporting these children rarely consider the potentially traumatic impact. Many believe anticipated death may be easier. The shock of sudden death produces great fear and confusion and prevents loved ones from saying their goodbyes, thus presenting greater challenges in coming to terms with the death.

This narrow view ignores the many emotional and logistical strains put on young children experiencing the impending death of a loved one. Along with these strains come intrusive images of the physical decline of their loved one. The very anticipation of the death may cause adverse psychological consequences for the child. The child may feel helpless because of his inability to change the dreaded outcome.

Children with a dying parent usually experience a great sense of terror and insecurity. Coupled with the fear of losing his parent comes the issue of "who is going to take care of me after the death?" Some surviving spouses of the dying parent are extraordinarily thoughtful in helping the child cope. They recognize that the very concept of death is extremely frightening to the child. They use verbal

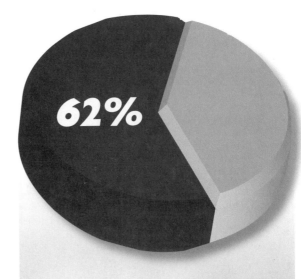

"62% of marriages will end in divorce within two years after the death of a child."

– Catholic Family Services and Lutheran Family Services

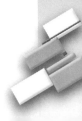

reassurance and physical presence to comfort and guide. Many parents however, preoccupied with their dying spouse, struggle to handle parenting duties and fail to help the child grapple with the impending death. Thus the child is left on his own to cope with a situation adults find extremely depressing.

Stressors for Children with a Dying Parent

- The physical, mental, and emotional decline of the dying parent
- Fear of the unknown – "who will care for me?"
- Loss of the sense of the world as an orderly, safe place
- Fear of own emotional reactions at the time of death
- Surviving parent is physically and emotionally unavailable
- Guilt – not being able to help or tolerate spending time with the dying parent due to physical, mental, and emotional decline.

Past Experience

In my past experience working with Hospice, I have experienced two extremes in children as they attempt to cope with a dying parent:

- *Those who don't want to, or refuse to spend time with the dying parent.* This reaction most probably stems from not being able to face the impending death and the physical, mental, and emotional decline of their dying parent. Guilt develops around the desire of not wanting to be around the parent.
- *Those who feel like they have to be with their dying parent every available moment.* They display not only tolerance, but an extreme sense of responsibility to "be there" for their dying parent. If the child gets too caught up in the situation and doesn't take a break to care for themselves and be a "normal" child, the heaviness of the situation can bring on stress, guilt, depression or other unhealthy behaviors.

Helping Children Through Anticipatory Grief

Adults who guide children through this traumatic process need to be extraordinarily thoughtful and keenly sensitive to the child's needs and fears.

Children with a dying parent usually experience a great sense of terror and insecurity.

The adult must recognize that the very idea of the death of a parent is frightening to the child. Both verbal reassurance and physical presence of the caring adult is crucial. Honesty with sensitivity is of paramount importance. The surviving parent must be able to distinguish positive exposure to the dying parent from exposure that could produce fearful memories, possibly causing elements producing future trauma.

In October of 1997, my father was dying in the critical care unit of our local hospital. I offered to take our son, Jeff, then 11 years old up to the hospital to see his grandfather for very possibly the last time. Jeff responded with a look of terror and went into his bedroom, sat on his bed, and started to cry. I went into the room and sat next to him, putting my arm around him and purposely staying silent. After a short time, Jeff looked up at me and said "I feel very bad about not wanting to go. I want to remember Grandpa the way he was when he was healthy and not the way he looked while he was dying." I responded by telling him he did not have to go and he didn't have to feel bad as this is a very sad time for all of us. I gave him an option. I said, "If you want to go to the hospital with me, you can sit in the waiting room in case you change your mind. If you do change your mind, you can just walk up to Grandpa's room. I promise I will not try to convince you to make a decision either way. I will respect your feelings. You have my word." I sensed a feeling of relief in Jeff. He said he wanted to drive with me to the hospital. As we entered the hospital, he took a seat in the waiting room as I took the elevator to my father's room on the 6th floor. As I entered the room I grabbed his hand and gave him a hug. As I took a step back to sit down, I saw my father's face light up as he peered behind me. As I turned to see what lit up his face, I saw Jeff enter the room. He hugged his grandpa and told him he loved him. My father died a short time later.

Jeff has thanked me several times for not insisting he go see his grandpa one last time. Jeff made the decision for himself, and to this day feels good about the decision he made. He thanks me most of all for empowering him to make a decision, being sensitive to his fears, and impressing on him that I would respect whatever decision he made. As he put it, "I offered him a choice about being exposed to his dying grandfather, but remained involved in the decision."

Conclusions

The greatest time of need for the child who must face the impending death of a loved one is at the time of diagnosis. Most people feel it is right after the death (which is indeed a critical time); however, experience and research prove otherwise. Separation anxiety occurs at the time of diagnosis as the child contemplates living in a world without his dying loved one. Secondary stress is common as the child will witness the grief and despair of his surviving family members. I strongly suggest that the child be adequately prepared for the time of death in an age-appropriate manner. The thoughtful surviving parent should invite the child to share his fears and give him choices around exposure to the dying loved one. However, the surviving parent should remain involved by guiding the child's decision and not insisting on what the feel is right at the moment. In many cases, guilt will manifest in the child as he knows he wasn't a perfect child, at times causing the dying loved one distress. The caring adult must be ready to dispel guilt feelings and help the child focus on the many good things he has done and reassure him that he is indeed a good child.

We cannot assume that anticipatory grief is easier than a sudden death. Although both situations are different and may present different issues, they are equally challenging in helping children to heal, regain hope, and learn again to love life.

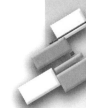

Sudden Death in the Family

Two Sisters Die in Accident

For many years, my wife and I have been close friends with a very loving couple who did a magnificent job raising their four children. The care and respect that each family member has for each other was clearly evident to us. One evening, two of their daughters were driving home from a school dance when a drunk driver ran a blinking red light which resulted in his slamming into the side of their vehicle. The collision killed both girls. This couple and their remaining two children went through a period of time (about the 4th to the 24th month) where they were almost totally torn apart emotionally. Each surviving family member was in so much pain that they couldn't reach out to each other and pull together. Frankly stated, the father refers to this time period for his family as "hell." Although you never totally get over a tragedy such as this, the family is back on the road to resolution after many extremely difficult struggles caused by the tragedy.

Colleague's Son Completes Suicide

A colleague of mine for eight years had a family of five children. His wife is a very wonderful, caring and loving mother. When my wife and I were dating, we said to each other that we wanted to be parents like this couple. Our goal was to raise a family as nice and caring as their family. Prior to our meeting this couple, they lost their second oldest son in a car accident. This family made it through their struggles that followed, but shared with us the many difficult times they had. One such struggle was communication within the family. Each family member was grieving in his or her own way and was unaware that this is okay. However, because each family member was unaware of this being okay, they judged each other based on their displays or non-displays of grief. Each member was either offending the others or afraid to offend the others and totally withdrew into their grief. Thus, instead of this family pulling together, they were pulling apart. Ten years to the date of this boy's death, their youngest son, Valedictorian of his class, well liked and respected, completed suicide. This was a total shock for all. I am compelled to think, but I don't know for sure, can an unresolved grief issue have been a cause of this horrible tragedy? My wife and I can only describe this family as the best of families. This family is going through another period of great suffering and pain. I have lunch with them quite often in their home. They have shared with me how difficult it is for them to reach to their surviving children because of their own pain, and how each one of them is grieving in their own unique way.

A Mother's Statement

Another story I wish to share comes from a mother who lost a son 20 years prior to being a guest speaker in my "Christian Perspective on Death and Dying" adult Sunday School class. This lady made a statement that I will never forget. She said, "After the death of my son, for roughly two years, the only energy I had was used up by rolling out of bed in the morning and getting dressed. I was in so much pain and had so little energy I could not possibly help my two remaining children with their grief."

Under Stress

The family is indeed under a great deal of stress at this time. The book "Mick Harte Was Here" by Barbara Park is a must read for anyone who wants a clear picture of what the death of a child does to a family. The story is about a boy named Mick Harte who was killed in a bicycle-automobile accident. It is narrated by his surviving sister, who is ten months older than Mick. It helps all who read the story to see the great turmoil families are in after the death of a loved one. After Mick's death, the family rarely ate meals together and, due to the difficulty of their pain, avoided each other all together. My experience in dealing with matters such as this leads me to believe that this story is a very common portrayal of the American family who has lost a loved one to death. This book is also a good reading project for the language arts teacher to use with upper elementary or lower middle school students.

In Conclusion–
The Point of these Stories

I share these stories with you to not only describe the turmoil, lack of communication, guilt and "cocooning syndrome" going on in the family after a death occurs, but also to stress the critical role you may have in helping the surviving children. Another good read is found in Alan Wolfelt's book, "Healing the Bereaved Child." The opening chapter is a parable about a wise old gardener who discovers a weak-looking seedling growing outside of his garden in rocky soil. The gardener assists the seedling, but is careful to give just enough care for the seedling to survive and blossom. This story is an excellent analogy for the caring adult as she guides the child through the grief process. If you have the opportunity to read this story, you need to take note of what the gardener did *not* do in caring for this forlorn seedling. You will notice that the gardener only intervened when the seedling was threatened by the frost or other elements that could have been fatal to this young plant. He didn't protect in the day-to-day hassles. He did not pass on his coping skills to the seedling. He helped the seedling develop its own coping skills.

A Substitute for the Deceased

A very important point that needs to be stressed at this time is in working with a grieving child. A relative, teacher, family friend, etc., should not attempt to become a substitute for a deceased parent. This, in many cases, destroys the relationship you have with this child. Grieving children many times will perceive the "substitute parent" as controlling and resist. This resistance can lead to a breakdown in the relationship, and as I have witnessed in many cases, a rejection of the adult by the child. There is a major difference in filling voids a child may have as a result of losing a parent and attempting to become a substitute for the parent. Voids which can be filled may include a fishing trip, a ball game, attendance at the grieving child's school play, etc. The caring adult must be aware of this difference.

What you have in your heart is more important than what you have in your head.

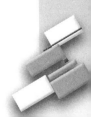

You Are Important

The point of this chapter is that you can play an extremely important role in assisting a child grieving the loss of a sibling or parent. If the rest of the family members are in so much pain and turmoil, they likely cannot reach to the grieving child. If they can't reach to this child, who will? You may say, "I need more courses in psychology or grief and bereavement." The classes may help. However, like I have stated before, what you have in your heart is more important than what you have in your head. Ninety-five percent of the time when your heart is right so will be the things you do in these situations. This book is written to help you with the other 5%. A simple hug, a listening non-judgmental ear, a "thinking of you" card or a liaison for the child between his teacher or surviving parent are a few of the many simple yet important things you can do. You don't have to have all the answers. I have learned that grieving children don't expect you to have all the answers. Remember, they need your comfort and support more than they need your advice.

What About Counseling?

Many times adults try to get the child into counseling as soon as possible. In working in these situations for many years, I have come to three conclusions:

1 People think that professional counseling can fix the child.

2 Many adults just don't want to deal with the tragedy themselves. They realize that reaching out to the child will force them to deal with issues they themselves don't want to deal with.

3 Some people feel it is the best thing to do at the time.

Although the first two reasons are obviously wrong, the third reason can be wrong as well. According to Dr. Joel Robertson, a well-respected psychiatrist, "In most cases, the greater need of the child at the time of tragedy and shortly after is the comfort and care of familiar faces rather than a professional." If the child can't yet feel his pain because he is still in the shock or denial stage, can counseling be effective? It is my experience that counseling has better results once the child can feel pain from the tragedy. Many adolescents in my support groups over the years have shared with me that they "could not remember the funeral of their deceased loved one." Some have shared they "can't remember anything for months after the tragedy." Many experts describe this as the "fight or flight" syndrome. In a great majority of these cases, the data shows that counseling at this time is ineffective. There is no doubt that in most cases, the professional counselor will have an important role, but the adult should not use the professional counselor as an excuse to back away and wash his hands of the situation.

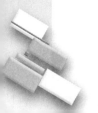

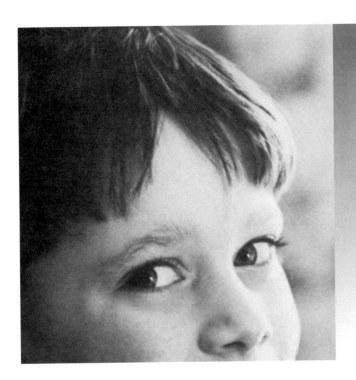

If they don't have you, who do they have?

Backing Away

Six years ago I had a young adolescent boy in my advisory group who, upon arriving home from school one day, found his mother dead on the kitchen floor. She shot herself to death. This young adolescent was assigned to my caseload by our school principal. After two years of sharing and building a quality relationship with this young man, plus some gentle nudging, I convinced him to go to a therapist. I made the referral and then made a critical mistake. Thinking I would be interfering, I backed away from seeing this boy on a regular basis. When I did see this boy, he gave me an indication that therapy was not going well. Upon calling the therapist, I found out why. The therapist stated that I should not be backing away. She said that I had two years of working experience with him and I needed to still be involved if the therapy was going to be effective. I learned a lesson from my mistake: even with the best counselor, therapist or psychologist, the grieving child still needs a caring adult to listen, guide and comfort him. The referral to a professional is no excuse to back away from the situation. If they don't have you, who do they have?

Chapter 6

Reintegrating the Child in School

Chapter Six
Reintegrating the Child in School

Imagine this situation. You're an elementary teacher and upon arrival at school one morning, you're informed that one of your student's father died the night before in a car accident. Then you find out that it is one of your students you highly enjoy having in class. You remember talking to her father and how smart and caring he was. This is a real prize of a family.

In a few minutes you will have to face the class and inform them of what happened. What will you say to them? How do you explain the unfairness of it all? How do you help the students be a support to the bereaved student? How do you reintegrate this student back to the classroom upon her return? Are there school guidelines for you to follow in this situation? In this chapter we will attempt to address these important issues.

The Role of the School Crisis Team

If your school and/or community has a well-established, trained crisis team, you will be in a much better situation to deal with the tragedy and to help your class work through the tragedy. If the school staff is traumatized by a particular tragedy, the community crisis team (such as police, fire department, local hospitals, etc.) can allow them to step back and get a handle on the situation while care is being provided for the students. The community crisis team should not be taken advantage of, however, by school staff stepping back and just choosing not to deal with the situation themselves. Many students are offended by this situation. Remember, students prefer to talk to people with whom they have established relationships.

You most likely would have been notified before you came to school by a call from your crisis phone chain. A staff meeting would be called for all staff who feel that their students will be impacted by this tragedy before the students arrive at the school the day following the incident. At this meeting, you will prepare for student questions and be given an announcement to be read to the class. A presentation by the crisis team family liaison will be given to present the facts, with permission from the family, to announce the death to the students. Announcements over the PA are totally inappropriate in this situation. The staff will be made aware of crisis rooms for students who may need extra help and instruction on how to get students to the crisis rooms. Classroom discussion guidelines will also be given to the staff and discussed. Information about funeral arrangements will be given. Staff sign-up sheets will be passed out for duty at the funeral home during visitation. For more concise information, plus sample announcements, letters home to parents, classroom discussion plans, staff meeting agendas and much more, you may consider my book, *Confronting Death in the School Family* (Published by National Center for Youth Issues). You can order a copy by calling (989) 249-4362, by e-mail griefrecovery@chartermi.net, or visit our website at www.griefrecovery.ws. Another valuable website is that of the Robertson Research Institute at www.robertsoninstitute.org.

Goals for the School

The school should have three goals when a tragedy such as the death of a student, staff member or family member of a student or staff member occurs.

1 Acknowledge the death honestly – Make sure the family liaison secures permission to announce the death at school from the family of the deceased.

2 Allow children and staff to ventilate – Many times the need for the staff to ventilate is overlooked. If the staff is given this opportunity, chances are that they can be a more effective support to the students.

3 Offer an outlet for the children's desire to help.

Normal or Abnormal Grief

At the beginning of the grief process, it is difficult to distinguish between normal and abnormal grief behavior. Usually, abnormal grief is demonstrated by extreme behavior. The following table includes typical normal and abnormal grief behaviors.

Normal	Abnormal
Responds to comfort and support	Rejects comfort and support
Uses play to express grief	Resists play
Connects depressed feelings with death	Doesn't relate feelings to life events
Often open and angry	May not directly express anger
Still experiences moments of joy	Projects a pervasive sense of doom
Caring adults can sense a feeling of chronic sadness and emptiness	Projects hopelessness and emptiness
May express guilt over some aspect of the loss	Has overwhelming feelings of guilt
Self-esteem temporarily impacted	Deep loss of self-esteem

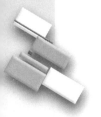

In discussion with parents, if it has been decided that the child can benefit from counseling, the child should be told so with compassion and understanding. The last thing the child needs to feel is that something is wrong with him. It may be appropriate to explain to the child that just as there are doctors to help with broken bones, there are caring people who can help in dealing with grief.

Hindrances to Children's Grief

Many factors can delay, distort or hinder the grief process. Therese Rando, an authority on grief in children, identified 14 factors that can make grieving harder for children who have experienced the death of a loved one. The first four factors directly relate to the death of a parental figure.

1 The surviving parent's inability to mourn

2 The surviving parent's inability to tolerate the pain of the child and allow the child to mourn

3 Fear about the vulnerability of the surviving parent and the security of self

4 Ambivalence towards the deceased parent

5 The lack of security associated with a caring environment

6 The lack of a caring adult who can stimulate and support the mourning process

7 Confusion about the death and one's part in it

8 Unchallenged "magical thinking"

9 An inability to put thoughts, feelings and memories into words

10 Issues of adolescence that exacerbate normal conflicts in mourning

11 Cognitive inability to accept the finality and irreversibility of the death

12 Lack of opportunities to share feelings and memories

13 Instability of family life after the loss

14 Reassignment of an inappropriate role and responsibilities

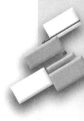

These factors may contribute to the reason why many children either suppress their grief or have delayed grief reactions. Young children look to adults to show them how to cope with the problems of life. The closest adults in a child's life can have a great impact in helping the child recognize a loss, understand when one is grieving, and identify and express feelings in appropriate ways.

The first day back in school after the death of a classmate is a very crucial day for students and staff alike, especially young students.

What Students Can Do

Besides making sympathy cards and writing condolence letters to their grieving classmate, group discussions should take place. These discussions can be led by the classroom teacher and should be about how they may be a support to their classmates. Invite the students to share. You will gain valuable insight from the students into the world of this grieving child. Giving students the opportunity for input helps them feel like they are an important part of the process in helping their classmate. Discuss the student's return with the class. Emphasize that the student has just experienced a great loss and will need a long time to adjust. Help the students think through how they will interact with the grieving student. Encourage them to be as normal as possible. Talk about helping the student feel like part of the class, as she was before the tragedy. Help the student feel welcome, but do not make a big fuss. Get back to a regular schedule as soon as you feel it is appropriate. Children find security in routines.

The Student's Return to School

When the student returns to class, welcome the student back and acknowledge the loss. It is usually a good idea to mention the name of the deceased person. In doing so, you will personalize their loss and ease their fear that their deceased loved one will not be forgotten. Quickly help the student reengage with the class. Let the student and the class know (through your actions) that life goes on. Carry on as usual. If the student breaks down, do not draw any attention to her. Have an activity planned that does not require teacher direction and then quietly comfort the student. The student should know that the teacher is there to help in any way possible. Offer the child a private place within the school to gather her composure.

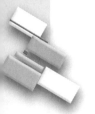

Specific Ideas for Elementary Students

The following is a list of ideas that the elementary classroom teacher may use to help when a child is grieving over the loss of a parent, sibling or other significant person in her life:

- Let the grieving student be the teacher's helper for the day.

- Provide the child with an opportunity to speak with a respected adult such as their teacher from the previous year, a favorite custodian, cafeteria worker, physical education teacher, principal, etc.

- Help the child express his/her feelings by working with art materials.

- Do not cause the student to feel "singled-out" or awkward with an open classroom, teacher or other group discussion of the personal loss in the presence of the student.

- Do not force the child to talk about the death. Most children will do so in their own way and time.

- A group hug from the whole class.

- Encourage classmates to be a support system.

The Death of a Classmate

The first day back in school after the death of a classmate is a very crucial day for students and staff alike, especially young students. The first order of the day should be to announce the death and help students process what happened through guided discussion, preferably led by the classroom teacher. A condolence letter from the entire class can be constructed with input from students, guided by the teacher. The students can then put together a book of poems or nice stories about the student who died. Encourage students to express their feelings in various ways to the deceased student's family.

Specific Activities Students Can Do

Before I get into specific activities about what students can do, I wish to mention some things they should *not* do. I don't feel that students should make a shrine out of the deceased student's locker or desk. Other students may have to use the desk during different class periods or use the locker the following year. Also, I don't think students should make a bulletin board in honor of the deceased student. Sooner or later, the bulletin board has to come down. I confess that I have done all three things in the past and

> The first order of the day should be to announce the death and help students process what happened through guided discussion, preferably led by the classroom teacher.

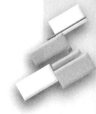

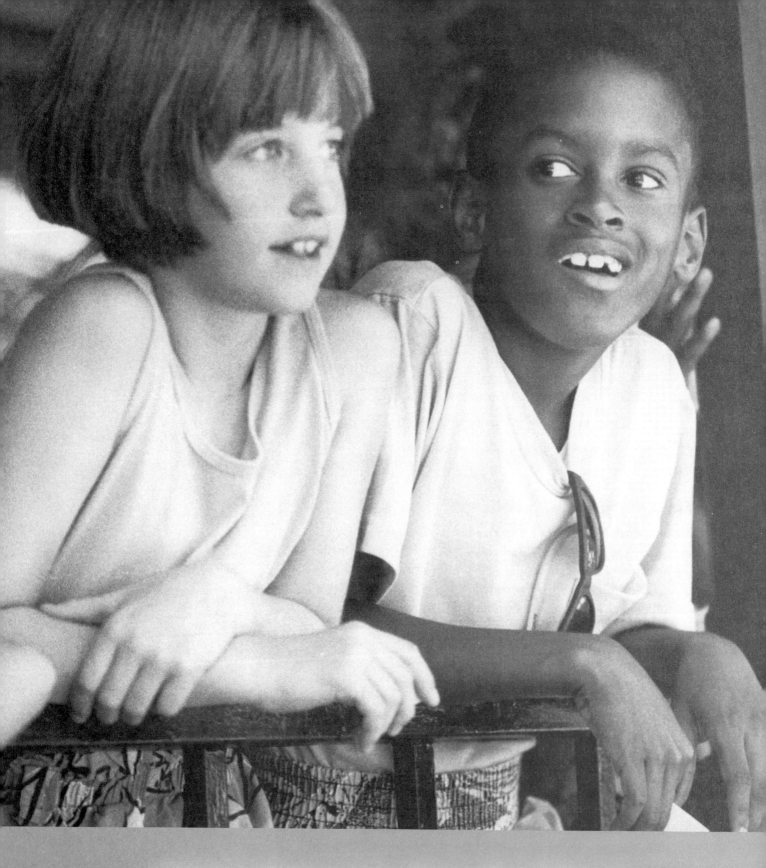

Get back to a regular schedule as soon as you feel it is appropriate. Children find security in routines.

admit that they are mistakes. If students so insist on making a bulletin board or shrine of the locker or the desk, set clear limits on when these shrines will come down. If these projects include letters to the deceased, poems, etc., explain to the students that they will be given to the deceased's family once they are taken down.

As we admitted our mistakes and looked for alternative activities, we have discovered a few very good ones. The following is a list of these alternatives:

- **A bulletin board display for visitation at the funeral home** – (*It is a good idea to have the family liaison clear this with the deceased's family first.*) Have students bring in pictures of activities with the deceased. Make sure students put their names on the back of the pictures so you can easily return them after the funeral. With the help and input of the students, use the pictures and other artwork or letters to make a display board. Place the display board at the funeral home where students can see it before they enter the chapel to view the deceased. The board helps to calm and place the students at ease by giving them something that is personal or familiar as they first enter the funeral home. Also, it may stop some students from expressing emotions which may be perceived as inappropriate by adults and other students by making the deceased a part of their lives. Most funeral directors are very willing to work with school personnel to make this happen.

- **Make a treasure box memorial** – An adult needs to oversee this project as well to make sure all things students bring are appropriate. Provide an appropriate-sized box. Have students bring stuffed animals, pictures, poems, songs, artwork, a letter to the deceased or anything that will cultivate a pleasant memory or be a fitting tribute. Have students present this to the parents after the wake service at the funeral home, during the luncheon after the funeral, or at some other appropriate time. The parents can keep the box forever and pass it down their family tree as they grow old.

- **Design and have T-shirts printed in honor of the deceased** – You may wish to sell the shirts with proceeds going to a memorial scholarship fund or other appropriate memorial activity.

I want to stress that we have done all of the above (the display bulletin board for the funeral home, treasure box memorial and scholarship activity) and claim that these three activities were much more appropriate and successful in getting students involved, while relieving the stress of when to take the bulletin board down or when to "de-shrine" the desk or locker.

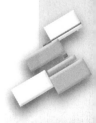

Appendix

"Thinking of You"
Information Sheet

Your Name _____

Name of Deceased _____

Date of Death _____

Parent _____ *Sibling* _____ *Grandparent* _____

Godparent _____ *Close Friend* _____ *Aunt/Uncle* _____ *Significant Person* _____

Deceased's Birthday _____

Parents Wedding Anniversary _____

Your Birthday _____

Days that are especially difficult for you during the year:

_____

_____

_____

_____

_____

_____

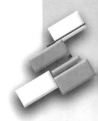

A person who I loved very much has died.

Use the balloons below for journaling. If you wish to write more than the space allows, you may continue journaling on an extra sheet of paper.

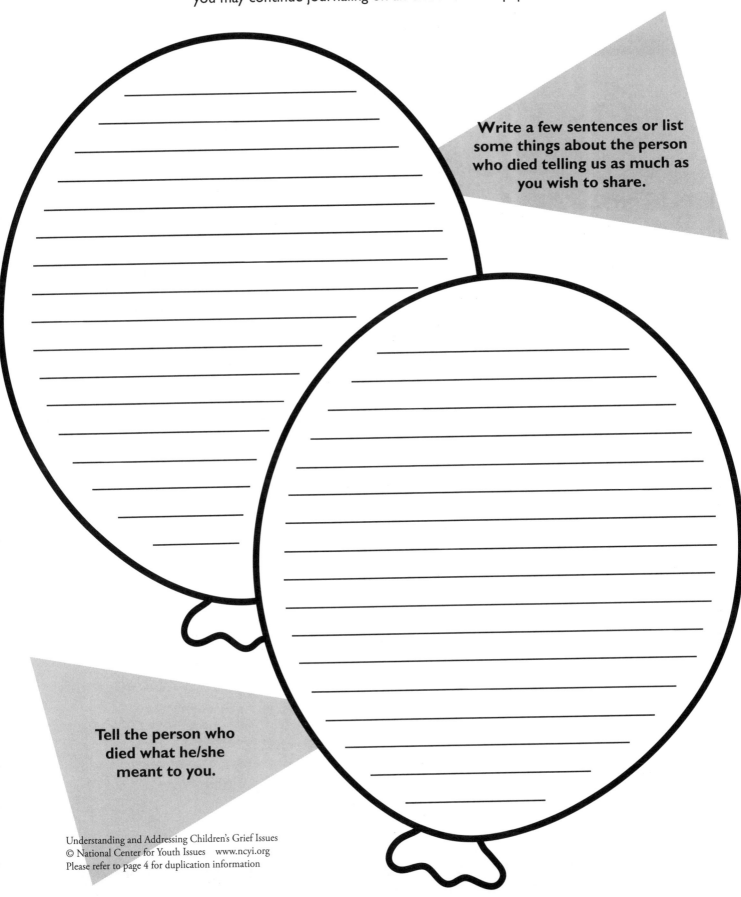

Write a few sentences or list some things about the person who died telling us as much as you wish to share.

Tell the person who died what he/she meant to you.

A person who I loved very much has died.

Color the picture below. Or, thinking of things you liked to do together, you can draw your own picture in the frame below of you and your loved one who died. You may wish to do both.

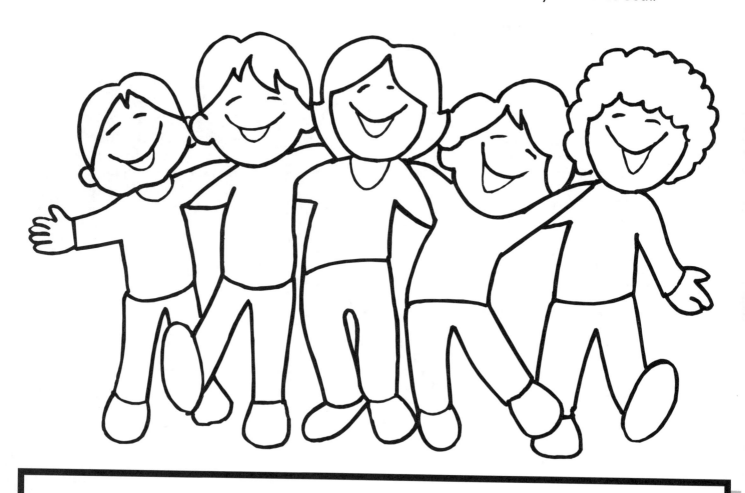

We had fun together, and I miss that.

Using the spaces provided, write a few sentences or make a list of things you and
your loved one who died did together. If you wish to write more than the space allows,
you may continue journaling on an extra sheet of paper.

Things we enjoyed.

**Our favorite things
we did together.**

**Our funniest time
together.**

We had fun together, and I miss that.

Color the picture below. Or, thinking of fun things you did, you can draw your own picture in the frame below of you and your loved one who died. You may wish to do both.

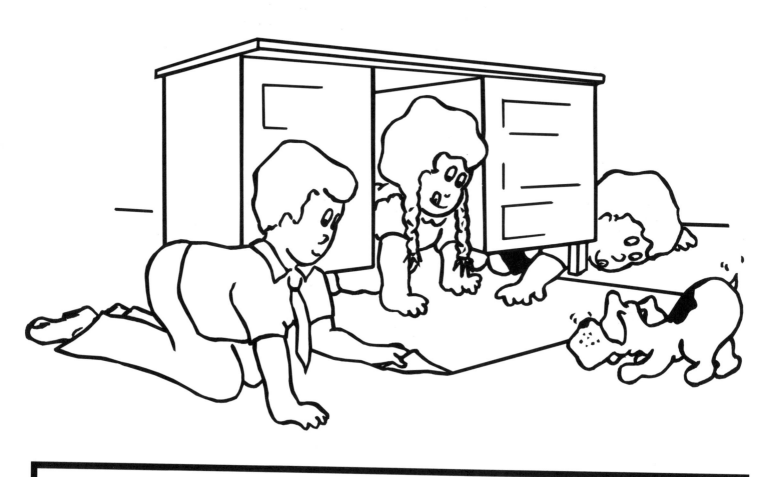

You are special, and I want to remember you.

Write a few sentences or make a list of things you remember about your loved one who died. If you wish to write more than the space allows, you may continue journaling on an extra sheet of paper.

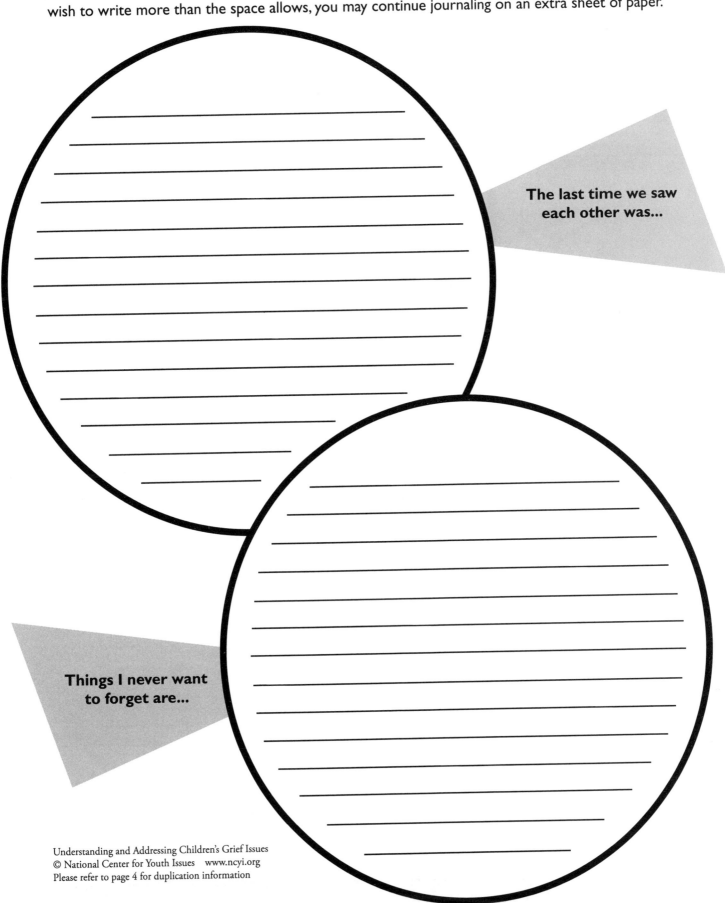

The last time we saw each other was...

Things I never want to forget are...

You are special, and I want to remember you.

Color the picture below. Or, thinking of things you remember, you can draw your own picture in the frame below of you and your loved one who died. You may wish to do both.

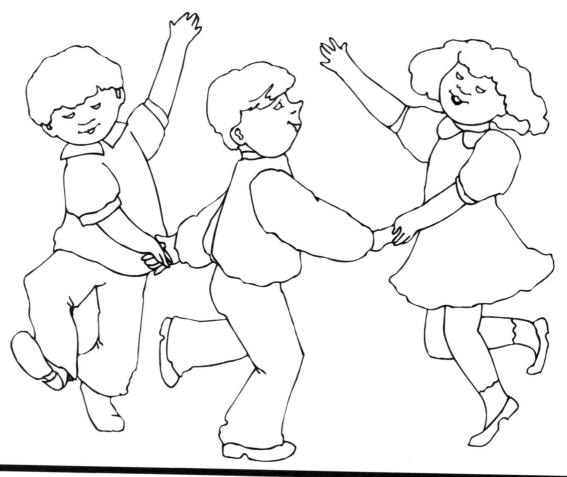

The day you died.

Write a few sentences or make a list about how and when
your loved one died. If you wish to write more than the space allows,
you may continue journaling on an extra sheet of paper.

**This is what I know
about when and how
you died.**

**These are my thoughts
about when and how
you died.**

The day you died.

Color the picture below. Or, thinking of things that happened the day your loved one died, you can draw your own picture in the frame below. You may wish to do both.

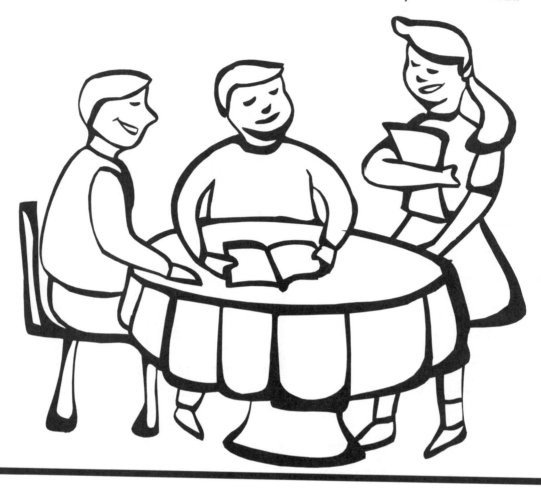

How I felt when I found out you died.

Write a few sentences or make a list about your feelings the day your loved one died. If you wish to write more than the space allows, you may continue journaling on an extra sheet of paper.

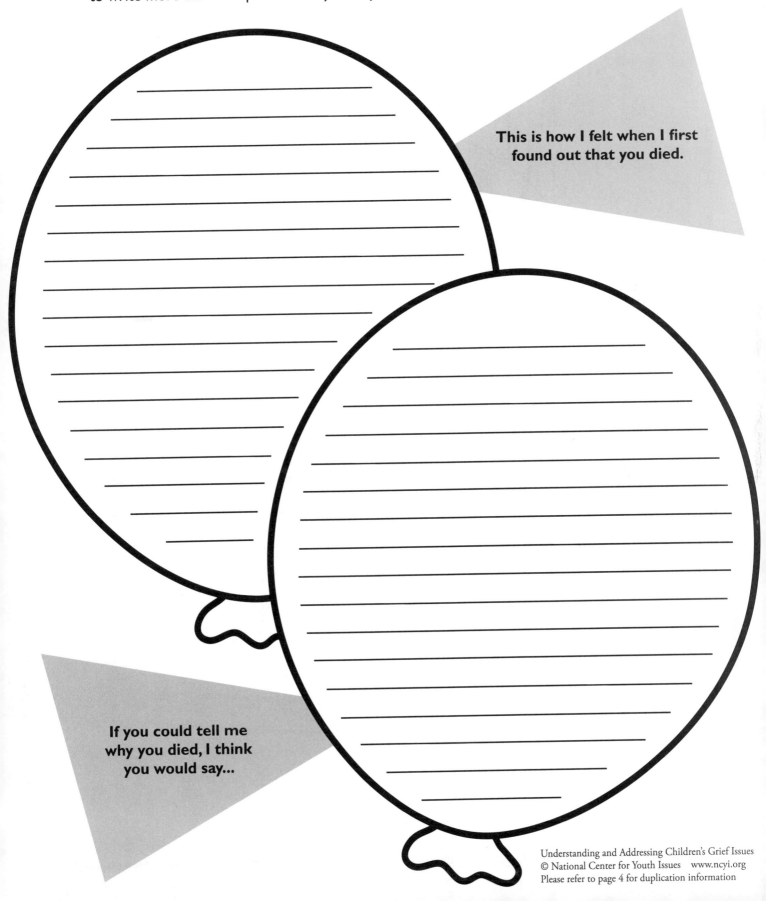

This is how I felt when I first found out that you died.

If you could tell me why you died, I think you would say...

How I felt when I found out you died.

Color the picture below. Or, thinking of how you felt when you discovered your loved one had died, draw your own picture in the frame below. You may wish to do both.

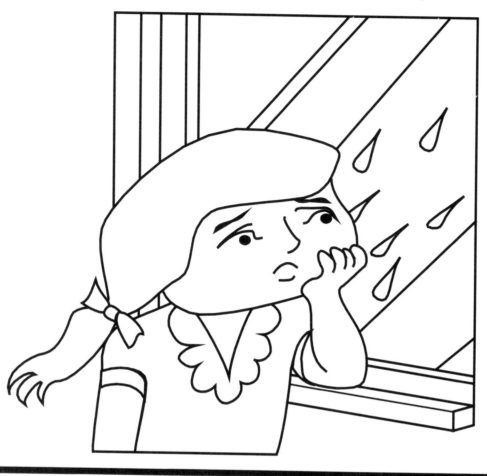

Your tombstone.

Think about what you would want everyone to know about your loved one. What made them so special to you? Then, on the tombstone image below, write what you would have printed on your loved one's tombstone so everyone would understand how special they were to you.

Drawing/Coloring Activity Six

Your tombstone.

In the space below, draw what you'd like your loved one's tombstone to look like.
Be creative. You can design the tombstone any way you like so everyone will understand
how special your loved one was to you.

How I feel now.

Write a few sentences or make a list about how you feel since your loved one died. Your feelings may range from anger to sadness to feeling that everything is unfair and you're lonely. If you wish to write more than the space allows, you may continue journaling on an extra sheet of paper.

I feel angry or sad because...

This is so unfair because...

I feel alone because...

How I feel now.

Finish the face below by drawing the mouth, nose, etc.
Try to make the face show how you feel inside since your loved one has died.

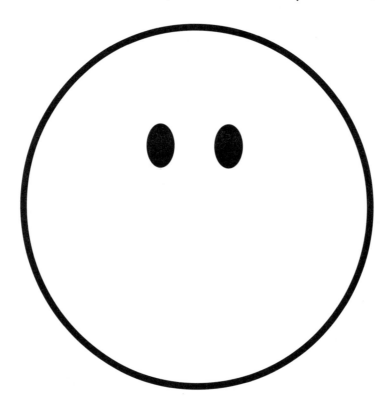

In the space below, draw a picture showing how you think others think you feel
since your loved one has died.

Fundamental Steps for Grief Survival
Helpful Hints for Caring Adults for Grieving Children

1. Recognize the loss – for a while you are numb. It has happened. Try not to avoid it.

2. Bear with the pain. You are hurting, admit it. To feel pain after a loss such as yours, is normal.

3. You are a beautiful, worthwhile person – you are much more than the emotional wound you are presently feeling.

4. Give yourself time to heal – believe that you will heal.

5. Heal at your own pace. Never compare yourself to another grieving person.

6. Be gentle with yourself. You have suffered an emotional wound, so treat yourself with care.

7. Good eating habits are important.

8. Suicidal thoughts may occur. They are a symptom of pain. If you feel that they are getting out of control, ***SEEK HELP AT ONCE!!!***

9. It is okay to feel anger. Most everyone gets angry at the loss of a loved one. Channel your anger wisely.

10. Give yourself praise. You are a deeper person with a wider perspective on life.

11. Expect relapses. There will always be certain things that trigger sadness again. This is normal.

12. Crying can be a cleansing and healthy release.

Note: The above is a short list. We encourage you to add to this list as you work with grieving children.

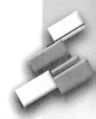

Parental Release Form

I _____, the parent of _____

    ☐   **DO** give my permission for my child to participate

    ☐   **DO NOT** give my permission for my child to participate

        in a Grief Support Group, established by _____.

Parents/Guardians signature _____

Principal signature _____

                        Date: _____

cc: Principal's Confidential File/Superintendent

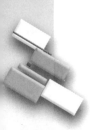

Valuable Resources

As I stated in the Forward section of this book, there is a wealth of very good and helpful resources concerning children and grief. The following list has been constructed for your convenience in locating them. Please note that because of the wealth of information, this list is not a complete list and many fine resources may not be listed.

A Child Remembers – by Enid Samuel Traisman, M.S.W.

This work is an outline to a journal the caring adult and grieving child can work through together. It gives good structure to the caring adult who may be hesitant about how to address the loss with the grieving child.

And God Cried Too – by Marc Gellman

This is a story about two angels, Gabe and Mikey. Mikey is Gabe's intern who is being trained to be a guardian angel through various life experiences, mostly lessons centered on grief. Reading this work is an excellent learning opportunity for the child caregiver as well as the child. Another must read.

Beautiful – by Susi Gregg Fowler

An insightful story about a young boy who is taught to grow a garden by his uncle, who is dying from a terminal disease. Uncle George must go to a faraway hospital for treatment. While away, the young boy plants a garden. Uncle George dies, but the gift he imparts to the young boy helps him to see the beauty in life.

Healing the Bereaved Child – by Alan Wolfelt

This book can serve as the Bible from A to Z for the caring adult wishing to understand and comfort the grieving child. Analogies are drawn between a veteran gardener (caregiver) and a seedling (grieving child) that are very enlightening and easy to apply. Activities and organizations are also included. A must read for anyone who wishes to offer support and comfort to children affected by the loss of a loved one.

How I Feel – by Alan Wolfelt

This is a coloring book for young grieving children in which the pictures represent many of the issues young children will go through when grieving the death of a loved one. This is a great opportunity for the adult to color alongside the grieving child, allowing the child to express his feelings in the way kids do best.

Mick Harte Was Here – by Barbara Park

This story is about what happens to a typical family after the death of a child. Mick Harte is killed in a bicycle-automobile accident. The story about what happens to his family after the death is narrated by his sister. Reading this book will give you a clear picture of the series of painful adjustments a family experiences after the death of a child.

My Mommy Has Cancer – by Carolyn Stearns Parkinson

A valuable resource in explaining cancer to a young child. It focuses on the loving care he receives from adults in his life. It is obvious to the reader that this work is created through great love and concern for children.

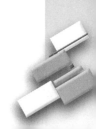

Talking With Young Children About Death – by Fred Rogers

This pamphlet is an extremely valuable resource to help parents in talking about death with their children. Difficult issues are explored and explained with the gift of sensitivity that made Mr. Rogers highly admired and respected.

Tear Soup – by Pat Schwiebert and Chuck DeKlyen

This is a very touching story about an elderly lady, Grandy, who experienced a loss. She cooks her unique batch of ingredients into her own grief process and shares them with her grandson. This is great lap reading material or story time material for young elementary or preschool children.

That Summer – by Tony Johnston

A touching story about two young brothers in which one of them, Joey, falls critically ill. It is very encouraging how Joey's family pulls together, especially when informed that Joey will die. That Summer was a season of family, of life and of love. Recommended for preschool and early elementary children.

When Dinosaurs Die – by Laurice Kransney Brown and Marc Brown

This is a very clear and sensitive guide geared toward the young child on understanding death. Another outstanding piece of work great for lap reading. This book will stimulate many worthwhile discussions between the caring adult and grieving child.

Where is Grandpa? – by T.A. Barron

A beautifully illustrated book which helps a young child who lost his grandfather focus on the good memories. Another great lap-reading opportunity which will stimulate quality discussion between the caring adult and the grieving child.

Why Did She Have to Die? – by Lurlene McDaniel

A touching story about a woman who struggles to cope with the death of her sister. Great reading for the upper elementary or lower middle school literature class

Young People With Cancer: A Handbook for Parents

Printed by the U.S. Department of Health and Human Services, this work does an excellent job of serving parents and family members of young cancer patients. It is a concentrated effort in the area of coping with childhood cancer. It also contains many important insights from the young cancer patient and his parents.

Other Recommended Resources

Daddy's Promise – Cindy Klein Cohen

A Child's Guide Through Grief – Alexis Cunningham

Help Me Say Goodbye Activities – Janis Silverman

If Nathan Were Here – Karen Jerome

I'll Always Love You – Hans Wilhelm

I Know Someone Who Died Coloring Book – Connie Manning

Remembering Mama – Dara Dokas

The Return of Rex and Ethel – Linda Gercey

Gentle Willow: A Story for Children About Dying – Joyce Mills

Don't Despair On Thursdays: Children's' Grief Management Book – Adolph Moiser

After the Funeral – Jane Loretta Winsch

Badger's Parting Gifts – Susan Varley

Everett Anderson's Goodbye – Lucille Clifton

I Miss You: A First Look at Death – Pat Thomas

Waterbugs and Dragon Flies: Explaining Death to Children – Doris Stickney

Where's Jess – Joy Jackson

The Three Birds: The Story for Children About the Loss of a Loved One – Bryan Mellonie

Muddles, Puddles, and Sunshine – Winston's Wish

Although this list is certainly incomplete, it is my wish that it can assist you in acquiring quality reference materials for you to better love, care and gently guide the child through these difficult situations.

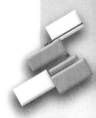

References

1. National Center for Health Statistics, Atlanta GA: Centers for Disease Control and Prevention.

2. Wolfelt, Alan, *Healing the Bereaved Child*, 1996, Companion Press.

3. Grollman, Earl, Death: *A Practical Guide for Living*, 1974, Boston Beacon Press.

4. Rando, T.A., *How to Go On Living When Someone You Love Dies*, New York, Boston Books

5. Gellman, Marc, *And God Cried Too*, 2002, Harper-Trophy

6. Kushner, H., *When Bad Things Happen to Good People*, 1981 Avon Books

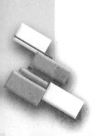